Delicious and Nutritious Keto Recipes

Simple, Affordable, Irresistible, Easy, and Healthy Ketogenic Diet Recipes

Debra Leo

Disclaimer

The information in this book is for educational purposes only. It should not be taken as a direct advice from medical care personnel. The advice from your physician remains the best source of information. Therefore, always seek medical advice from your doctor to ascertain if your body or health condition allows for keto diet recipes like the ones in this eBook.

All the recipes in this book are approved by dieticians. The recipes are tasty and healthy and can give you the best results a keto diet can offer. But they may not be suitable for all individuals without some modifications.

We made sure that you get the best recipe you can find but consultation from your doctor is required before you start. It is your responsibility to evaluate and confirm the information in my ebook with other sources. Get the involvement of your physician or any qualified medical health care professional before you embark on the keto diet recipe journey.

TABLE OF CONTENTS

Recipe 1

Almond Lemon Cake Sandwiches

Ingredients

¼ teaspoon of salt

¼ teaspoon of liquid stevia

½ teaspoon of apple cider vinegar

½ teaspoon of baking soda

½ vanilla extract

½ almond extract

1 teaspoon of cinnamon

1 tablespoon of coconut milk

1 tablespoon of lemon juice

¼ cup of butter

¼ cup of coconut flour

¼ cup of Honeyville almond flour

For garnishing: 2 tablespoons of crushed pistachios

For garnishing: zest ½ lemon

Sandwich Icing

1 teaspoon of red food coloring

2 tablespoon of heavy cream

4 tablespoon of butter

2 ounces of cream cheese

¼ cup of powdered erythritol

How to prepare the recipe

1. Heat the oven up to 325F.
2. Sift and carefully mix almond flour, cinnamon salt, coconut flour, and baking soda.
3. Put in one place eggs, vanilla extract, lemon juice, erythritol, vinegar, coconut milk, melted butter, food coloring, and stevia.
4. Add the wet ingredients to the dry ones and mix with a hand mixer until everything is fluffy.

5. Divide the butter and place on muffing top pan. Bake for about 18 minutes.

6. Carefully remove the pan from the oven and allow it to cool on the rack for up to 10 minutes.

7. Slice the cakes in half and let them fry in butter until crispy.

8. Allow the crispy cakes to cool on the rack again

9. Mix everything together: heavy cream, butter, powdered erythritol, cream cheese until fluffy.

10. Color the recipe by adding food coloring.

11. Add icing in-between cakes and form a sandwich.

12. Use pistachios and lemon zest to garnish.

The above ingredients can make up to 10 cakes in total. Each cake including icing will have:

Calories: 180
Fats: 17.5 grams
Protein: 2.8 grams
Carbs: 1.8 grams

Recipe 2

Inside Out Bacon Burger

Ingredients

¼ teaspoon of Worcestershire

¼ teaspoon of onion powder

½ teaspoon of salt

¾ teaspoon of soy sauce

½ teaspoon of black pepper

½ teaspoon of minced garlic

1 ½ teaspoon of chopped chives

2 slices of chopped bacon

200 grams of ground beef

How to Prepare the Recipe

1. Cook chopped bacon in a cast-iron skillet until crisp. Cook well, remove it and place it on paper towel. Separate and save grease in a different container.

2. Add together 2/3 chopped bacon, ground beef, and all spices and mix in a large bowl.

3. Mix spices and meat and form them into 3 patties.

4. Heat 2 tablespoons of bacon fat on a cast iron, and once the fat is hot, add patties.

5. Allow cooking for about 5 minutes on either side until cooked according to your taste.

6. Remove and cool for at least 3 minutes. Serve with cheese, onion, and extra bacon

The above ingredients can make up to 1 serving of 3 patties made up of:

Calories: 649

Fats: 51.8 grams

Protein: 43. 5 grams

Carbs: 1.8 grams

Recipe 3

Bacon and Mozzarella Meatballs

Ingredients

½ teaspoons of kosher salt

½ teaspoons of onion powder

2 teaspoon of minced garlic

1 teaspoon of pepper

2 large eggs

1/3 cup of crushed pork rinds

¾ cup of mozzarella cheese

4 slices of bacon

1 ½ pound of ground beef

How to Prepare the Recipe

1. Heat the oven ahead up to 350F.
2. Carefully cut the bacon into cube-like pieces.

3. Add ground beef, eggs, ground pork rinds, and spices to bacon.

4. Mix well until they form meatballs.

5. Roll meatballs into circular shapes. Place on a foiled baking tray.

6. Put in oven and bake for 40 or 45 minutes.

7. Use a spoon to take out ½ tablespoon pesto sauce for each meatball.

8. Serve bacon and mozzarella meatballs.

The above ingredients can make up to 24 meatballs.

Each meatball contains:

Calories: 128

Fat: 9.4 grams

Protein: 10.1 grams

Carbs: 0.7 gram

Recipe 4

Bacon Infused Sugar Snap Peas

Ingredients

½ teaspoon of red pepper flakes

2 teaspoon of garlic

3 tablespoon of bacon fat

½ lemon juice

3 cups of sugar snap peas

How to Prepare the Recipe

1. Add 3 tablespoons of bacon fat and allow it to reach the smoking point.
2. Add garlic, reduce the heat, and allow for 1 or 2 minutes.
3. Put sugar lemon juice and snap peas. Cook for 1 or 2 minutes.
4. Remove from pan and serve.

5. Garnish recipe with lemon zest and red pepper flakes.

The above ingredients will yield 3 servings in total.

Each serving will have:

Calories: 147

Fats: 13.3

Protein: 1.3 grams

Carbs (net): 4.3 grams

Recipe 5

BBQ Pulled Chicken

Ingredients

1 teaspoon of red boat fish sauce

1 teaspoon of cayenne pepper

1 teaspoon of cumin

2 tablespoons of chili powder

1 tablespoon of soy sauce

1 tablespoon of liquid smoke

2 tablespoon of spicy brown mustard

2 tablespoon of yellow mustard

¼ cup of organic tomato paste

¼ cup of chicken stock

¼ cup of red wine vinegar

¼ cup of erythritol

1/3 cup of salted butter

6 skinless, boneless chicken thighs

How to Prepare the Recipe

1. Mix all the ingredients, excluding chicken thighs and butter.

2. Set a slow cooker and cook frozen or fresh chicken thighs. Pour sauce afterward.

3. If you can't wait, add butter and turn the cooker low and allow for 7-10 hours.

4. If you are home, cook for 2 hours on low heat. Add butter and increase heat, and allow for 3 hours more.

5. Once the chicken is cooked, shred with two forks.

6. Mix sauce and cook in high heat for 45 minutes in an open-top pan. This should reduce the sauce.

7. Sprinkle coarse sea salt, curry powder, and chili pepper over it and serve.

The above ingredients should yield 4 servings in total, and each serving will contain:

Calories: 510
Fats: 30 grams
Protein: 51.5 grams
Carbs: 2.3 grams

Recipe 6

Buffalo Chicken Strips

Ingredients

1 teaspoon of onion powder

1 teaspoon of garlic powder

2 teaspoons of pepper

2 teaspoons of salt

1 tablespoon of chili powder

1 tablespoon of paprika

2 eggs (large)

3 tablespoons blue cheese crumbles

3 tablespoons of butter

¼ cup of olive oil

½ cup of hot sauce

¾ cup of almond flour

5 chicken breasts with ½ inches pounded thickness

How to Prepare the Recipe

1. Heat the oven ahead.
2. Add together salt, garlic powder, pepper, onion powder, chili, and paprika in a ramekin.
3. Pound chicken breasts to reach ½ thickness, and then cut in half.
4. Mix spice and sprinkle 1/3 on the chicken. Turn over the chicken and sprinkle the same quantity.
5. Mix 1/3 of the spice mix and almond flour together.
6. Break and whisk 2 eggs in a bowl
7. Did seasoned chicken in the spice. Dip in the almond flour until both sides coat well.
8. Place each on a rack on top of the foiled baking sheet.
9. Bake chicken for up to 15 minutes.
10. Remove from oven and switch oven to broil. Pour 2 tablespoon of olive oil on the chicken.

11. Broil the chicken for 5 minutes and flip in the process. Pour the remaining olive oil and broil for an additional 5 minutes.
12. Add together 3 tablespoons of butter and 1/2 cup of hot sauce in a saucepan.
13. Serve with blue cheese crumbles and hot sauce slathering.

The above ingredients should yield 9 chicken servings in total.

Each serving will have:

Calories: 683

Fats: 54 grams

Protein: 41 grams

Carbs: 4.8 grams

Recipe 7

Recipe KetoProof Coffee

Ingredients

1 tablespoon of heavy cream

1 tablespoon of coconut oil

1 tablespoon of unsalted butter

Seasoning of choice

How to Prepare the Recipe

1. Use a measuring cup to make coffee and pour it into a large container.
2. Measure 1 tablespoon of butter and add it in the coffee.
3. Add a tablespoon of coconut oil into the container of coffee.
4. Measure a tablespoon of heavy cream to make it creamy.
5. Add cinnamon, allspice or nutmeg, and liquid stevia if you want to.

6. Mix well with a hand blender

The above ingredients should yield 1 serving of keto proof coffee, which contains:

Calories: 273
Fats: 30 grams
Protein: 0 gram
Carbs: 1 gram

Recipe 8

Chai Spice Mug Cake

Ingredients

¼ teaspoon of vanilla extract

¼ teaspoon of cardamom

¼ teaspoon of clove

¼ teaspoon of ginger

¼ teaspoon of cinnamon

2 tablespoons of Honeyville almond flour

½ baking powder

7 drops of liquid stevia

1 tablespoon of NOW erythritol

2 tablespoons of butter

How to Prepare the Recipe

1. Add together all room temperature ingredients and mix them in a mug.

2. Put the mug content in a microwave and turn high for about 1 minute 10 seconds.
3. Turn the cup upside down and knock it round to ease removal.
4. Add whipped cream and a sprinkle of cinnamon on top if you like it that way.

The above ingredients should yield 1 serving in total, which is:

Calories: 493
Fats: 42 grams
Protein: 12 grams
Carbs: 4 grams

Recipe 9

Bacon Cheddar Explosion

Ingredients

2 teaspoon of Mrs. Dash table seasoning

1 or 2 tablespoons of Tones Southwest chipotle

4 to 5 cups of raw spinach

2 ½ cups o cheddar cheese

30 slices of bacon

How to Prepare the Recipe

1. Heat the oven to about 375F before you start.
2. Weave bacon by placing 15 pieces vertically, 12 pieces horizontally, and the remaining ones to fill in horizontally as well.
3. Add seasoning mix to the bacon.

4. Add cheese to bacon with 1 ½ gap between edges.

5. Put in spinach, press down to compress.

6. Carefully roll the weave and make it tight so nothing falls through. Some cheese may fall out though but that's no problem.

7. Add seasoning here if you like it that way.

8. Get a foil sheet and add sprinkle plenty of salt on it.

9. Place the baking sheet on a cooling rack and put the bacon there.

10. Bake the bacon for 1 hour or 1 hour 10 minutes. This should make your bacon crisp when finished.

11. Cool for 10 or 15 minutes before taking it off the rack.

12. Slice the bacon into smaller pieces and serve.

The above ingredients should yield 3 servings in total.

Each serving will have:

Calories: 720

Fats: 63 grams

Protein: 54 grams

Carbs: 4.9 grams

Recipe 10
Cheddar Chorizo Meatballs

Ingredients

1 teaspoon of kosher salt

1 teaspoon of chili powder

1 teaspoon of cumin

2 eggs (large)

1/3 cup of crushed pork rinds

1 cup of tomato sauce

1 cup of cheddar cheese

1 ½ chorizo sausages

1 ½ pound of ground beef

How to Prepare the Recipe

1. Heat the oven ahead if preparation time.

2. Break sausage into smaller pieces to mix well subsequently.

3. Add eggs, cheese, spices, ground pork, and ground beef to the sausage pieces.
4. Mix all ingredients until they form meatballs.
5. Shape them into circles and put on a foiled baking tray.
6. Bake the balls for 30 or 35 minutes. They should be cooked by then, but if they don't, bake until cooked.
7. Add tomato sauce on the top with a spoon, and serve.

The above ingredients should yield 24 medium-size meatballs in total.

Each will have:
Calories: 115
Fats: 7.8 grams
Protein: 9.9 grams
Carbs: 0.8 gram

Recipe 11

Cheesy Scrambled Eggs

Ingredients

1 teaspoon of chopped chives

1 ounce of cheddar cheese

2 tablespoons of butter

2 eggs (large)

Seasoning and spices of your choice

How to Prepare the Recipe

1. Add butter to pan and heat on the oven.

2. When butter melts, break 2 large scrambled eggs.

3. Cook the egg slowly and touch them at intervals at most two times.

4. Add any salt, hot sauce, chives, or any seasoning of your choice.

5. Add cheese to the recipe and mix it together.

The above ingredients should yield 1 serving only, which will have:

Calories: 453

Fats: 43 grams

Protein: 19 grams

Carbs: 1.2 gram

Recipe 12

Cheesy Spinach

Ingredients

½ teaspoon of pepper

½ teaspoon of salt

½ of Mrs. Dash

3 tablespoons of butter

1 ½ cup of cheddar cheese

How to Prepare the Recipe

1. Heat the pan on the stove and add butter.
2. When the butter melts, add spices and spinach, and allow spinach to wilt.
3. After wilting the spinach almost completely, shred the cheese on top and allow it to melt.
4. Once the cheese melts, serve the food.

The above ingredients should yield 2 servings in total.

Each serving will have:
Calories: 446
Fats: 47 grams
Protein: 24 grams
Carbs: 4.8

Recipe 13

Chicken Roulade

Ingredients

Pepper

Salt

38 grams of halloumi cheese

¼ teaspoon of minced garlic

¼ lemon zest

2 ¼ teaspoons of olive oil

½ tablespoon of pesto

1 chicken breast

How to Prepare the Recipe

1. Pat chicken breast until no moisture remains, and pound till 1/8 inches.

2. Combine 1 ¼ tablespoon of olive oil and pesto. Mix and spread on chicken.

3. Add garlic, pepper, lemon zest, and salt to the chicken.

4. Slice the halloumi and add to chicken.

5. Roll up chicken breast and then tie with butcher's string.

6. Heat oven up to 450F.

7. Use cast iron and heat high 1 teaspoon of olive oil.

8. Sear both chicken sides until they turn brown.

9. Bake until juice comes out.

The above ingredients should yield 1 serving, which will have:

Calories: 478

Fats: 31 grams

Protein: 53.3 grams

Carbs: 2.5 grams

Recipe 14

Buffalo Strip slider

Ingredients

For almond flour buns

8 drops of liquid stevia

½ teaspoon of apple cider vinegar

1 teaspoon of paprika

1 teaspoon of southwest seasoning

1 teaspoon baking soda

4 tablespoons of butter

3 tablespoons of parmesan cheese

2 eggs (eggs)

¼ cup of flaxseed

1/3 almond flour

Chicken filling

2 (two) leftover buffalo chicken strip

How to Prepare the Recipe

1. Heat oven before preparation.
2. Use a large bowl to mix all the ingredients together.
3. Put the butter in the microwave and melt.
4. Add vinegar, butter, eggs, and stevia to the mixture.
5. Carefully mix everything.
6. Spread mixture evenly on 8 muffins slotted in a pan.
7. Bake for 15 or 17 minutes.
8. Allow to cool for 5 minutes, and cut all the buns in halves.
9. Combine slider with buns and buffalo chicken strip.

The above ingredients should yield 8 buns servings in total, but only 2 buns are enough for a serving.

Each serving will have:

Calories: 625

Fats: 51 grams

Protein: 34.8 grams

Carbs: 4.3

Recipe 15

Bacon Cheddar and Chive Biscuit

Ingredients

¼ teaspoon of Mrs. Dash

Pinch of salt

1 tablespoon of chopped chives

1 tablespoon of packed shredded white cheddar

1 tablespoon packed cheddar

1 tablespoon of almond flour

2 slices of cooked bacon

½ teaspoon of baking powder

2 tablespoons of almond flour

1 egg

2 tablespoons of butter

How to Prepare the Recipe

1. Combine all room temperature ingredients and mix them in a mug.
2. Put in a microwave and turn high for 1 minute 10 seconds.
3. Turn the mug upside down and bang it until the recipe comes out.
4. Allow for 3 or 4 minutes to cool if you want it that way.

The above ingredients should yield 1 serving, which will have:

Calories: 573
Fats: 55 grams
Protein: 24 grams
Carbs: 5 grams

Recipe 16

Cinnamon and Orange Beef Stew

Ingredients

1 bay leaf

¼ teaspoon of sage

¼ teaspoon of rosemary

½ teaspoon of fish sauce

½ teaspoon of soy sauce

½ teaspoon of ground cinnamon

¾ teaspoon of minced garlic

¾ teaspoon of fresh thyme

¼ of orange juice

¼ of orange zest

1 tablespoon of coconut oil

¾ cup of beef broth

½ pound of beef

How to Prepare the Recipe

1. Slice the meat to about 1-inch cube and add orange zest.
2. Use a cast-iron skillet and heat coconut oil until it smokes.
3. Add pepper and salt to meat and put the meat in the skillet one after the other.
4. When the beef turns brown, take out the last batch from the skillet. Add vegetables, and cook for 1 or 2 minutes.
5. Pour orange juice to make the pan de-glazed. Add other ingredients except for thyme, sage, and rosemary.
6. Allow it to cook and then move all the ingredients to a crockpot.
7. Cook for 3 hours on high heat.
8. Add remaining ingredients/spices to the crockpot, and cook for 1 or 2 hours.

Note: You can double or quadruple the quantity if you want to save some for another day.

The above ingredients should yield 1 serving, which will have:

Calories: 649

Fats: 44.5 grams

Protein: 53.5 grams

Carbs: 1.9 grams

Recipe 17

Coffee and Red Wine Beef Stew

Ingredients

2 teaspoons of garlic

Pepper and salt

2 tablespoons of coconut oil

1 medium-size onion

2/3 cup of red wine

1 ½ cups of mushrooms

3 cups of coffee

2.5 pounds of stew meat

How to Prepare the Recipe

1. Cut the meat into small cubes and slices mushrooms and onions thinly.

2. Pour 3 tablespoons of olive oil into a pan and cook on a stove until it smokes.

3. Add seasonings (pepper and salt) to the beef, and brown it in small batches.

4. After that, remove the meat and use its fat to cook garlic, onion, and mushrooms.

5. Put beef stock, coffee, capers, and red wine together with vegetables and stir.

6. Combine the beef with the mixture and boil before turning the heat low.

7. Cover the pot and cook for about 3 hours.

The above ingredients should yield 4 servings in total. Each serving will have:

Calories: 755

Fats: 48.3 grams

Protein: 63.8 grams

Carbs: 4 grams

Recipe 18

Crispy Curry Rubbed Chicken Thigh

Ingredients

Pinch of cinnamon

Pinch of salt

Pinch of cardamom

1/8 teaspoon of coriander

1/8 teaspoon of chili powder

1/8 teaspoon of allspice

1/8 teaspoon of garlic powder

¼ teaspoon of paprika

¼ teaspoon of cumin

½ teaspoon of salt

½ teaspoon of tallow curry

1 tablespoon of olive oil

2 chickens (thighs)

How to Prepare the Recipe

1. Heat the oven before preparation.
2. Put all the spices and mix in a bowl.
3. Place the chicken thighs on a baking sheet foil.
4. Evenly rub olive oil on the chicken thighs.
5. Rub the mixture of spice all over the chicken thighs.
6. Bake the chicken thighs for 40 or 50 minutes.
7. Allow it to cool for about 5 minutes before you serve.

The above ingredients should yield 1 serving, which will have:

Calories: 555
Fats: 39.8 grams
Protein: 42.3 grams
Carbs: 1.3 grams

Note: If this is your week 4, make one extra meal of this recipe.

Recipe 19

Drunken Five Spice Beef

Ingredients

½ teaspoon of onion powder

1 teaspoon of cayenne pepper

2 teaspoon of cumin

1 teaspoon of salt

1 tablespoon of pepper

1 tablespoon of five-spice

2 teaspoon of minced ginger

2 tablespoons of soy sauce

3 tablespoons of reduced sugar ketchup

75 grams of raw spinach

135 grams of chopped broccoli

150 of sliced mushrooms

1 can of Coors Light or ½ cup of red wine

1 ½ pound of ground beef

How to Prepare the Recipe

1. Carefully chop the broccoli florets, garlic, and ginger.

2. High heat your ground beef on an iron cast.

3. Make all the beef brown before adding garlic and ginger.

4. Mix well, then add soy sauce, spices and broccoli and stir thoroughly.

5. Add 1 can of red wine or Coors light into the pan. Then put spinach and mushrooms and mix all.

6. When the spinach wilt, add your ketchup and serve.

The above ingredients should yield 4 servings in total. Each serving will have:

Calories: 515

Fats: 35 grams

Protein: 33.3 grams

Carbs: 6 grams

Note: if there are leftovers, put them in the freezer.

Recipe 20

Cheesy Frittata Muffins

Ingredients

¼ teaspoon of salt

½ teaspoon of pepper

2 teaspoon of dried parsley

1 tablespoon of butter

½ cup of cheddar cheese

4 ounce of bacon (chopped and pre-heat)

½ cup of Half n' Half

8 eggs (large)

Note: You can use any spice, sauces, or seasonings you like. You can add red pepper flakes, reduced sugar ketchup, or mayonnaise if you choose.

How to Prepare the Recipe

1. Heat your oven up to 375F.

2. Combine half n' half with eggs and mix until scrambled.

3. Fold in the spices, cheese, and bacon, and then add other ingredients at this point.

4. Rub butter on muffin tin, which should be up to 8 in number.

5. Fill each cup with the mixture up to ¾ of the cups.

6. Put them in the oven for 15 or 18 minutes, or until they are puffy has gold color on the edges.

7. Remove cups from the oven and allow them to cool for at least 1 minute.

8. Put in freezer, and heat one after the other when you want to serve subsequently.

The above ingredients should yield 8 servings in total. Each serving will have:

Calories: 205

Fats: 16.1 grams

Protein: 13.6 grams

Carbs: 1.3 gram

Recipe 21

Fried Queso Fresco

Ingredients

½ tablespoon of olive oil

1 tablespoon of coconut oil

1 pound of queso fresco

How to Prepare the Recipe

1. Slice the cheese into smaller cubes or rectangles.
2. High heat ½ tablespoon of olive oil, and 1 tablespoon of coconut oil in a pan.
3. Allow to smoke before adding cheese. Let it cook until turned brown and turn the other side and allow it to brown too.
4. Take out the pan and remove excess grease.

The above ingredients should yield 5 servings in total.

Each serving will have:

Calories: 243

Fats: 19.5 grams

Protein: 16 grams

Carbs: 0 gram

Recipe 22

Lemon Rosemary Chicken

Ingredients

1 teaspoon of kosher salt

½ teaspoon of dried ground sage

¾ teaspoon of dried rosemary

1½ teaspoon of fresh thyme

1 lemon

1½ teaspoon of olive oil

1½ of minced garlic

3½ boneless, skinless chicken thighs

How to Prepare the Recipe

1. Put ½ teaspoon of salt and garlic in a mortar.
2. Use a pestle to grind the two ingredients.
3. Carefully add oil while grinding, mixing, and turning it into the aioli.

4. Once it is done, dry the chicken and put in a bag with the aioli, making sure the chicken is coated well.

5. Soak the chicken in a marinade for between 2 – 10 hours.

6. Heat your oven up to 425 degrees.

7. Thinly slice a lemon and arrange slices on the baking pan bottom.

8. Place the chicken on the lemon slices.

9. Pick thyme leaves from their stem and add the thyme, sage, pepper, rosemary, and extra salt to the chicken.

10. Bake the entire mix for 25 or 30 minutes, or until the juiced flows out.

11. Take out the chicken and put pan drippings in a saucepan.

12. Boil the sauce and stir while boiling.

13. Reduce the heat to medium-low, stirring the sauce all the time until it reduces.

14. Use a spoon to spread the sauce on the chicken and serve.

The above ingredients should yield 1 serving, which will have:

Calories: 589

Fats: 40.5 grams

Protein: 47 grams

Carbs: 4.2 grams

Recipe 23

Keto Szechuan Chicken

Ingredients

½ teaspoon of minced ginger

½ teaspoon of Mrs. Dash table blend

1 teaspoon of red pepper flakes

2 teaspoons of pepper

2 teaspoons of salt

2 teaspoons of spicy brown mustard

1 tablespoon of red wine vinegar

1 tablespoon and 1 teaspoon of erythritol

2 tablespoons of chili garlic paste

3 tablespoons of coconut oil

4 tablespoons of organic tomato paste

½ cup of chicken stock

6 cups of spinach

1½ pounds of ground chicken

How to Prepare the Recipe

1. Add and mix tomato, garlic paste, soy sauce, ginger, and brown mustard in a ramekin.
2. Boil 3 tablespoons of coconut oil on medium-high heat.
3. Add salt and pepper to the chicken and cook in the heated oil until cooked through.
4. Break the chicken up into smaller pieces.
5. Put 2/3 of sauce to the mix and stir well.
6. Add spinach to chicken and allow it to wilt.
7. Add pepper and salt, red pepper flakes, and Mrs. Dash seasoning.
8. Add chicken stock, erythritol, red wine vinegar, and remaining 1/3 sauce.
9. Mix in well the spinach and spices.

10.	Bring the heat to low, cover the pan, and allow it to cook for 10 or 15 minutes.

The above ingredients should yield 3 servings in total.

Each serving will have:

Calories: 515

Fats: 38.3 grams

Protein: 63 grams

Carbs: 5.2 grams

Recipe 24

Not Caveman's Chili

Ingredients

1 teaspoon of Worcestershire

½ teaspoon of cayenne pepper

1 teaspoon of oregano

2 teaspoons of paprika

2 teaspoons of minced garlic

2 teaspoons of red boat fish sauce

2 teaspoons of cumin

2 tablespoons and 1 teaspoon of chili pepper

2 tablespoons of olive oil

2 tablespoons of soy sauce

1/3 cup of tomato sauce

1/3 cup of beef broth

1 medium-size green pepper

1 medium-size onion

2 pounds of stew meat

How to Prepare the Recipe

1. Cut half of the stew meat into smaller cubes and use the food processor to process to turn the other into ground beef.
2. Cut the onions and pepper.
3. Mix all spices together and make a sauce of them.
4. Fry the cubed beef in hot fat on a pan until t turns brown.
5. Move and place the pan of fried beef to a slower cooker.
6. Fry the ground beef in hot fat.
7. Do the same with the vegetables until onions become translucent.
8. Put everything so far on the slower cooker and mix.
9. Simmer the content for 2½ hours on high heat.

10.   Again simmer for 20 n94 30 minutes without covering the pan or pot.

Note: reduce the quantity of your chili pepper if you are not comfortable with it.

The above ingredients should yield 4 servings in total. Each serving will have:
Calories: 398
Fats: 17.8 grams
Protein: 51.8 grams
Carbs: 5.3 grams

Recipe 25

Omnivore Burger with Creamed Spinach and Roasted Almonds

Ingredients

1 teaspoon of red pepper flakes

1 teaspoon of cumin

½ tablespoon of Tone's Southwest chipotle seasoning

½ tablespoon of butter

½ tablespoon of heavy cream

1 tablespoon of cream cheese

2½ tablespoons of roasted almonds

2½ cups of raw spinach

¼ of bell pepper

¼ of onions

1 cup or 100 grams of sliced mushrooms

1 pound of ground beef

How to Prepare the Recipe

1. Heat the oven up to 450 degrees (convection) or 475 degrees (normal).
2. Put 100 grams of mushrooms, ¼ bell pepper and ¼ onions in a food processor until they are diced.
3. Put together diced vegetables, meat, and seasonings and mix well in a bowl.
4. Measure out 3 portions of burger patties of the meat mix.
5. Place the patties on a cooling rack on a baking sheet covered in foil. Add salt to it.
6. Sizzle a small amount of meat in a pan.
7. Put spinach and allow it to wilt with other ingredients such as red pepper flakes, salt, and pepper.
8. Add butter, cream cheese, heavy cream, and almonds and stir well.
9. Continue to cook the Recipe.

10.   Take out the burger from the oven after about 19 or 24 minutes.

Note: keep your eye on the cooking due to their ability to cook fast.

The above ingredients should yield 2 servings in total.

Each serving will have:
Calories: 562
Fats: 38.5 grams
Protein: 45.3 grams
Carbs: 4.8 grams

Recipe 26

Bacon Wrapped Pork Tenderloin

Ingredients

Pinch of dried sage

Pinch of cayenne

Pinch of black pepper

¼ teaspoon of dried rosemary

¼ teaspoon of liquid smoke

¼ teaspoon of minced garlic

¾ teaspoon of soy sauce

1½ teaspoon of sugar-free maple syrup

2½ teaspoons Dijon mustard

2½ of sliced bacon

½ pound of pork tenderloin

How to Prepare the Recipe

1. 1. Combine all dry and wet ingredients together to form a marinade.
2. Tap tenderloin until dry and put in Ziploc bag.
3. Pour the marinade into the Ziploc bag, rub on tenderloin, and put everything in the fridge for 3 or 5 hours.
4. Heat the oven up to 350 degrees.
5. Place the pork tenderloin on a foil baking sheet. Wrap it in bacon. Five slices should go into each tenderloin.
6. Bake the recipe for about 1 hour.
7. Broil the bacon for at least 5 minutes.
8. Use a foil to cover the tenderloin for 10 or 15 minutes.
9. Cut and serve the recipe.

The above ingredients should yield 1 serving, which will have:

Calories: 418

Fats: 20 grams

Protein: 54 grams

Carbs: 0.3 gram

Recipe 27

Red Spinach Salad

Ingredients

½ teaspoon of red pepper flakes

1½ tablespoons of parmesan cheese

2 tablespoons of ranch dressing

3 cups of spinach

How to Prepare the Recipe

1. Put spinach in a bowl, and drench in ranch.
2. Combine everything and mix it together.
3. Put red pepper flakes and parmesan.
4. Mix together and serve.

The above ingredients should yield 1 serving, which will have:

Calories: 208

Fats: 18 grams

Protein: 8 grams

Carbs: 3.5 grams

Recipe 28

Roasted Pecan Green Beans

Ingredients

½ teaspoon of red pepper flakes

1 teaspoon of minced garlic

½ lemon zest

2 tablespoons of parmesan cheese

¼ cup chopped pecans

2 tablespoons of olive oil

½ pounds of green beans

How to Prepare the Recipe

1. Heat the oven up to 450 degrees.

2. Add pecans to your food processor and grind until nicely chopped. Allow ground pieces to be both large and small.

3. Mix green beans, olive oil, lemon zest, red pepper flakes, parmesan

cheese, and minced garlic in a large bowl.

4. Bring foiled sheet and spread green beans on it.

5. Put the green beans in the oven for 20 to 25 minutes.

6. Allow to cool for at least 4 minutes and serve.

The above ingredients should yield 3 servings in total.

Each serving will have:

Calories: 182

Fats: 16.8 grams

Protein: 3.7 grams

Carbs: 3.3 grams

Note: freeze the leftovers for another day.

Recipe 29

Shrimp and Cauliflower Curry

Ingredients

¼ teaspoon of xanthan gum

¼ teaspoon of cinnamon

¼ teaspoon of cardamom

½ teaspoon of turmeric

½ teaspoon of coriander

½ teaspoon of ground ginger

1 teaspoon of paprika

1 teaspoon of cayenne

1 teaspoon of onion powder

1 teaspoon of chili powder

1 teaspoon of garlic powder

1 tablespoon of cumin

1 tablespoon of coconut flour

2 tablespoons of curry powder

3 tablespoon of olive oil

¼ cup of heavy cream

¼ cup of butter

1 cup of coconut milk

½ head medium of cauliflower

1 medium-size onion

4 cups of chicken stock

5 cups of raw spinach

24 ounces of shrimps

How to Prepare the Recipe

1. Combine all the spices on your list except xanthan.
2. Slice 1 medium size onion.
3. High heat 3 tablespoons of olive oil in a pan.
4. Add onion to the olive oil and cook till the onion is soft.
5. Put heavy cream, butter, spices, and xanthan in the oil, stir well, and allow for 2 minutes.
6. Add 1 cup of coconut milk and 4 cups of chicken broth and stir thoroughly and cover it for 30 minutes.

7. Add cut cauliflower and curry together and put in. Cover and allow it to cook for 15 minutes.

8. Bring shrimp and add to the curry. Cook for another 20 minutes.

9. Measure 1/8 xanthan gum and coconut flour and add to the mix. Stir well and cook for about 5 minutes.

10. After that, put in the spinach and stir to mix well. Allow cooking for another 5 or 10 minutes without cover.

The above ingredients should yield 6 servings in total.

Each serving will have:
Calories: 331
Fats: 19.5 grams
Protein: 27.4 grams
Carbs: 5.6 grams

Note: if this is your week 2, make double the quantity of the recipe.

Recipe 30

Simple Lunch Salad

Ingredients

¼ lemon zest

¾ teaspoon of curry powder

1 ½ teaspoon of Dijon mustard

1 or 2 tablespoons of parmesan cheese

2 cups of spinach

2 tablespoons of olive oil

Meat

How to Prepare the Recipe

1. Add together every wet ingredient and mix in a small bowl.

2. Add spinach and meat together in a bowl.

3. Pour the wet ingredients on the spinach and meat.

The above ingredients should yield 1 serving.

Recipe 31

Keto Snickerdoodle Cookies

Ingredients

2 tablespoons of cinnamon

¼ teaspoon of baking soda

1 tablespoon of vanilla

¼ cup of maple syrup

¼ cup of coconut oil

2 cups of almond flour

How to Prepare the Recipe

1. Heat the oven up to 350 degrees.
2. Combine together salt, baking soda, and almond flour.
3. Put in a separate bowl maple syrup, stevia, vanilla, and coconut oil and mix.
4. Combine wet and dry ingredients until they form a dough.

5. Mix together erythritol and cinnamon until they form a powder.

6. Roll the dough to form balls and roll the balls in the cinnamon mixture. Place the balls on a Silpat.

7. Grease bottom of a mason jar and use it to make the balls flat.

8. Bake the flattened balls for 9 or 10 minutes.

9. Remove from the oven and allow it to cool.

The above ingredients should yield 14 cookies in total.

Each serving will have:

Calories: 132

Fats: 12.4 grams

Protein: 3.4 grams

Carbs: 2 grams

Recipe 32

Low-Carb Spice Cakes

Ingredients

Spice Cakes

¼ teaspoon of ground clove

½ teaspoon of ginger

½ teaspoon of allspice

½ teaspoon of nutmeg

½ teaspoon of cinnamon

1 teaspoon of vanilla extract

2 teaspoon of baking powder

4 eggs (large)

5 tablespoons of water

½ cup of salted butter

¾ cup of erythritol

2 cups of Honeyville almond flour

Cream Cheese Frosting

½ lemon zest

1 teaspoon of vanilla extract

3 tablespoons of erythritol

2 tablespoons of butter

8 ounces of cream cheese

How to Prepare the Recipe

1. Heat the oven up to 350 degrees.
2. Mix sweetener and butter in a mixing bowl and make them cream smooth together.
3. Break 2 eggs into it and keep stirring.
4. Add the remaining two eggs and mix them together.
5. Grind all the dry spices and add them to the mix.
6. Put water into the mix and stir until creamy.
7. Take out your cupcake tray and fill it up to 3/4.
8. Put the cupcake in the oven for about 15 minutes.
9. While it's cooking, mix into cream your butter, vanilla, lemon zest,

sweetener, and cheese butter ready for frosting.

10.   Take out a cupcake from the oven, and allow it to cool for up to 15 minutes.

11. Add frost on them.

The above ingredients should yield 12 frosted cakes in total.

Each cake will have:

Calories: 283

Fats: 27 grams

Protein: 7.3 grams

Carbs: 3.3 grams

Recipe 33

Chicken and Bacon Sausage Stir Fry

Ingredients

½ teaspoon of red pepper flakes

2 teaspoons of minced garlic

2 tablespoons of salted butter

¼ cup of red wine

½ cup of Rao tomato sauce

½ cup of parmesan cheese

3 cups of spinach

3 cups of broccoli florets

4 chicken sausages

How to Prepare the Recipe

1. Cut 4 bacon and cheddar chicken sausages.
2. Boil water on the stove.
3. Put sausage in a pan and place on high heat.

4. Put broccoli in the boiling water, and cook for about 3 or 5 minutes.

5. Stir sausage until it is brown on each side.

6. Push the sausages on one part of the pan. Pour butter on the other side.

7. Add garlic to the butter and fry quickly for 1 minute.

8. Now mix together all the things in the pan.

9. Add broccoli.

10. Add tomato sauce, red pepper flakes, and red wine.

11. Put pepper, salt, and spinach, and allow it to cook.

12. Simmer for about 5 or 10 minutes.

13. Garnish it with fresh parmesan cheese and serve.

The above ingredients should yield 3 servings in total.

Each serving will have:

Calories: 451

Fats: 28.3 grams

Protein: 35.7 grams

Carbs: 7.3 grams

Recipe 34

Taco Tartlets

Ingredients

Pastry

2 tablespoons of cinnamon

¼ teaspoon of cayenne

¼ teaspoon of paprika

1 teaspoon of oregano

1 teaspoon of xanthan gum

¼ teaspoon of salt

5 tablespoon of coconut flour

1 cup of blanched almond flour

Filling

¼ teaspoon of cinnamon

1 teaspoon of Worcestershire

1 teaspoon of salt

½ teaspoon of pepper

1 teaspoon of cumin

2 teaspoons of garlic

2 teaspoons of yellow mustard

1 tablespoon of olive oil

2 tablespoons of tomato paste

3 stalks of spring onion

80 grams of mushrooms

400 grams of ground beef

1/3 cup of cheddar cheese

How to Prepare the Recipe

1. Put all dry ingredients for the pastry in a food processor.
2. Cut butter into smaller cubes and put in the food processor.
3. Make the dough crumbly, and add 1 tablespoon of cold water to make it pliable.
4. Freeze the dough for 10 minutes.
5. Use a rolling pin to roll the dough between two silpats.
6. Use a cookie cutter to cut out circles.
7. Put the cut circles into a whoopie pan.

8. Heat the oven up to 325 degrees.

9. Prepare your onions, mushrooms, and garlic.

10. Fry garlic and onions in olive oil.

11. Put mustard and tomato paste before ending frying.

12. Use a spoon to scoop ground beef into the tartlets.

13. Use cheese to cover the tartlets and bake for about 20 or 25 minutes.

14. You may choose to broil for 3 or 5 minutes before removing from the oven.

15. Allow cooling before removing pastries.

The above ingredients should yield 11 tartlets in total.

Each tartlet will have:

Calories: 241

Fats: 19.4 grams

Protein: 13.1 grams

Carbs: 1.7 gram

Recipe 35

Thai Peanut Chicken

Ingredients

Salt

Pepper

¼ teaspoon of cayenne pepper

¼ teaspoon of coriander

2 teaspoons of chili garlic paste

½ teaspoon of sesame oil

½ tablespoon of erythritol

½ tablespoon of coconut oil

1 tablespoon of rice vinegar

1 tablespoon of lemon juice

1 tablespoon of orange juice

2 tablespoons of soy sauce

¼ cup of chicken stock

1 cup of peanut butter

6 skinless and boneless chicken thighs

How to Prepare the Recipe

1. Rinse the peanuts, spin in a salad spinner to remove moisture.
2. Pat with paper towels until dry.
3. Put nuts in a food processor and blend to form a creamy substance.
4. Put erythritol and coconut oil in the creamy substance and blend more.
5. Except for cayenne, chicken, pepper, and salt, mix all the other ingredients.
6. Cut chicken thighs in cubes and add pepper and salt.
7. Pour 1 tablespoon of olive oil in pan and heat.
8. Once hot, add chicken.
9. Use a paper towel to pat out any remaining moisture.
10. Cook until chicken turns brown on each side.
11. Add peanut butter sauce and stir.

12. Add ¼ teaspoon of cayenne pepper, and pepper and salt.
13. Reduce heat to low and allow it to simmer for about 10 minutes.

The above ingredients should yield 2 servings in total.

Each serving will have:

Calories: 743

Fats: 53.5 grams

Protein: 70.5 grams

Carbs: 8.8

Recipe 36

Vanilla Latte Cookies

Ingredients

17 drops of liquid stevia

¼ teaspoon of cinnamon

½ teaspoon of kosher salt

½ teaspoon of baking soda

1½ teaspoon of vanilla extract

1 tablespoon and 1 teaspoon of coffee grounds

2 eggs (large)

1/3 cup of unsalted butter

1½ cups of Honeyville blanched almond flour

How to Prepare the Recipe

1. Heat the oven up to 350 degrees.

2. Add together baking soda, cinnamon, salt, coffee grounds, and almonds in a mixing bowl.

3. Put egg yolk and white in a separate bowl.

4. Use another mixing bowl to beat your butter.

5. Add erythritol to the butter and continue to beat it until white.

6. Mix the egg yolk with the butter and stir until smooth.

7. Pour half of your almond flour into the butter and stir to mix.

8. Put liquid stevia and vanilla extract, then pour the other half of almond flour and mix in.

9. Beat egg white until white.

10. Fold the egg white into the dough.

11. Separate cookies on cookie sheets, and bake for 12 or 15 minutes.

12. Remove cookies and allow them to cool on a rack for 10 to 15 minutes.

The above ingredients should yield 10 cookies in total.

Each cookie will have:

Calories: 167

Fats: 17.1 grams

Protein: 3.9 grams

Carbs: 1.4 gram

Recipe 37

Vegetable Medley

Ingredients

½ teaspoon of red pepper flakes

1 teaspoon of pepper

1 teaspoon of salt

2 tablespoons of minced garlic

2 tablespoons of pumpkin seeds

90 grams of spinach

90 grams of bell pepper

115 grams of broccoli

240 grams of baby belly mushrooms

6 tablespoons of olive oil

How to Prepare the Recipe

1. Dice, cut, and slice all the vegetables into small pieces.
2. Pour oil in pan and heat.
3. Add and fry the garlic in hot oil for 1 minute.
4. Put mushrooms and allow them to soak up oil.
5. After that, put in broccoli and mix it in well.
6. Allow the broccoli to cook for a few minutes.
7. Pour sugar snap peas and mix well.
8. Put bell pepper, pumpkin seeds, and spices and mix well.
9. When everything cooks, place spinach on the vegetables and steam.
10. When spinach wilt, mix well again and serve.

The above ingredients should yield 3 servings in total.

Each serving will have:

Calories: 330

Fats: 30.7 grams

Protein: 6.7 grams

Carbs: 7.7